FAREWELL TO MY COMPANION

Our Battle With Dementia

DIANA HUTTON

Copyright

Farewell To My Companion

Our Battle With Dementia

© Diana Hutton and HPEditions 2021
© cover design Diana Hutton and HPEditions 2021
Portrait on Front Cover by Angelo Resmini, 2016

**Categories: Biography, Personal Memoirs,
Family and Relationships, Ageing, Alzheimer's & Dementia**

All rights reserved under all international and Pan-American Copyright Conventions. By payment of the required fee, you have been granted the non-exclusive, non-transferable right to access and read the text of this book on screen. No part of this text may be reproduced, transmitted, downloaded, decompiled, reverse engineered or stored in any information storage or retrieval process in any form without the express permission of the publisher.
The moral rights of the author have been asserted.

Digital editions by HPEditions, June 2021 available everywhere
Print edition by HPEditions also available from most major retailers

Print edition ISBN: 978-0-6488380-9-8
Epub edition ISBN: 978-0-6488380-8-1
Kindle edition ISBN: 978-0-6451710-0-6

Length: 21,000 words

Published by HPEditions

CONTENTS

Eusebio (photo)	Frontpage i
Prologue	Frontpage ii
My Companion	1
Our Enemy	9
Santander Bay, September 2014 (photo)	19
Eusebio - Whiling away the hours in his garden (photo)	26
An Escapade	27
And the Days Go By	33
Catón, our beautiful cat, now deceased (photo)	34
Eusebio - On the lounge sofa beside Alba, February 2020 (photo)	36
Eusebio – with Diana, July 2020 (photo)	48
The Carer	49
Ambling	53
In our younger years (photo)	65
Medical Assistance	67
The Final Weeks	73

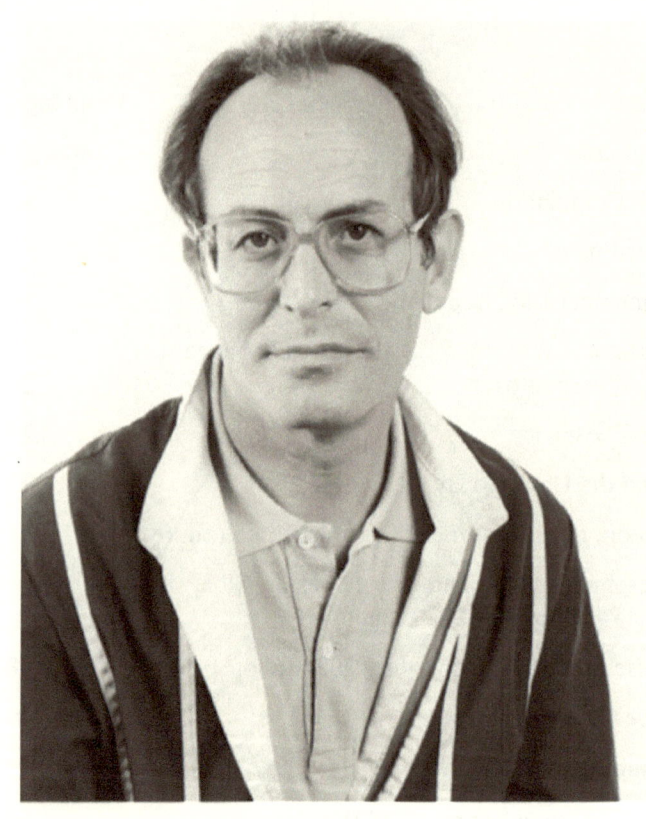

Eusebio

Prologue

It has not been my intention in this book to delve into the possible causes of dementia and in particular Alzheimer's Disease. Though it seems to be all around us, neither doctors nor scientists know very much about its causes, at least today, in the early years of the twenty-first century. These pages have been, above all, a personal memory exercise and putting my memories on paper has helped me to endure a situation which has in no way been easy.

No, I am not looking for sympathy. I fully accept having been the principal carer of my husband during his last years of illness. As far as I am concerned that is absolutely logical and, although it is one of the duties of marriage, it is a duty that is carried out with love, with a certain abnegation and, obviously, with many moments of frustration. As I explain below, I am not a nurse, neither am I a particularly patient person and I am certainly not a martyr. I have no desire to suffer for anything at all. However, all I realise is that the daily care of my husband fell within the range of my capabilities and I feel that I have done what I have done with pleasure, knowing that this final pathway is also part of life, part of the experience that one accumulates during life's journey.

I speak of enduring the situation. How did I endure it? Writing about it has been cathartic for me. Just as you can use the telephone or write messages to communicate with friends and family, I have been able to fill long hours writing this chronicle and, whether well or badly done, it has been like balm for my spirit, so often perturbed when seeing my life-time companion taking leave of me and the rest of his family. There is nothing sadder than being witness to someone you love profoundly who is gradually losing his mental faculties.

My Companion

What was my companion thinking about when he told me to *sew* the hole in the floor?

"Sew it up", he said.

"Sew what up?", I asked.

"That", he said.

"What is 'that'?"

"That!" he answered.

"That" was a large hole made to uncover some pipes that were leaking and it would have had to be filled with cement and stone tiles, something that he himself could have done easily had his mind been intact. It couldn't be sewn, but he was only aware that it had to be covered over. But why use the word "sew"? Did he say "sew" because I am a woman and, although I am not a seamstress, is this what he considered that women should do in life? When I say this, I am harking back to his roots, to his roots in a small Castilian village in León, where the men worked the land and the women looked after the house and cooked and mended the tears in their men's clothes. That was a long time ago, just after the end of Spain's Civil War, because although some women in Spanish villages still carry out those tasks, many of them, as in so many countries, have flown from the nest to move to the cities and to highly responsible jobs. The inhabitants of Castile are known in particular for their austere nature, for their nobleness and generosity and also because they are extremely hard-working. Life has changed, however, over the last fifty years. Yet for someone suffering from memory failure, the longer the time between a memory and the present, the easier it seems to remember. It is the present, or the near present, which disappears from their memories. It is why they constantly repeat the same question because they can't recall from one minute to the next what they have asked, nor the answer. They only know that something in their heads forces them to go over and over the same thing.

Eusebio was my companion and we were married almost fifty years. Easy to say. When I look back it seems to me that those years have passed as fast as a bird's flight. To be more specific, it is fifty-two years since I fell in love with his sensitive essays written while at the *Alliance Française* in Paris, back in the revolutionary days of France's May '68. Those early years in *Paris* were like a dream. I had come from Australia, on the other side of the world, where summer is winter and where it is hot at Christmas time, where the swans are black, not white, where the flowers are exotic and beautiful but have no perfume, a land of koala bears and kangaroos that carry their offspring inside a pouch for several months after their birth. They are known as marsupials and are a curiosity in the zoos of the cultured Europe. Australia was then a paradise of innocence, tucked away as it was on the other side of the globe, a land of opportunity, of good, easy living for many, of generous, happy-go-lucky souls who welcomed the outsider for what he was, without questions. And there were starting to be many outsiders back in the 1960s when I lived there. They were flooding in from Europe, Greeks and Italians above all, in search of a future, far from their troubled lands. They worked hard, bringing with them their culinary arts, their bright personalities, their attractive difference and they have all contributed to building the Australia of today. But there had been fewer immigrants from Spain, a few during the gold-rushes, a few more came to work on cane farms and some more in the late fifties after the end of the Civil War, but to Australians at that time, Spain was rather exotic. Perhaps it was these differences that attracted us to each other.

In Paris, I remember that Eusebio and I would walk for hours along the banks of the River Seine, talking, getting to know each other, turning our blossoming love into words, into ideas. We would go frequently to the theatre, sitting up "in the gods", the cheap seats, to see the plays of Beckett, Ionesco, of the exiled Spaniard, Fernando Arrabal. We used to read Simone de Beauvoir, Sartre and, in particular, Albert Camus. That was our Parisian adventure. We loved Paris even though we felt on the fringe of Parisian life. But then, we always felt that we tended to exist on the margin of mainstream life.

Eusebio in particular considered that he was only reluctantly accepted in Paris, because he formed part of the cohort of southern immigrants who, escaping fascism, had fled to France in search of money, a better life and who took on the most unpleasant, yet necessary, tasks which the French people no longer wanted to do. And some Parisians could be rather snobbish, even towards their provincial compatriots. But Paris was the heart of Europe, both for him as a Spaniard and for me as an Australian. I loved the majestic buildings lining the river, the cafés overflowing with clients nibbling on delicious croissants and crusty baguettes. The city had an aesthetic quality over and above that of London, at least for me. It seemed to be a just mixture of beauty and efficiency and I doted on hearing the French language around me. As for Eusebio, he considered at times that the Parisians had a superior air when treating foreigners, a certain tired boredom when they bothered to try to make the stranger understand their fluent dialogue. Also, being the often outspoken Spaniard he was, he found the French excessively polite and indirect. Or insincere? Yet it is right to say that France was better than Spain in those days because you could earn money, but he had left behind the blue skies, the sun, Spain's vast expanses of countryside, the happy voices of the people, all that which vibrated in his veins despite himself.

Did he, in 2020, recall anything from those years? He said he didn't, that he didn't remember our walks beside Paris' unforgettable river, that he didn't remember the theatre, or the company where he used to work, not in the offices but as a messenger. However, those must have been some of his most stimulating years because in Paris he could enjoy a freedom then only dreamed of in Franco's Spain. Years of theatre, of reading and, yes, of love. How could he forget them?

This is not the place, neither is it my intention, to offer an account of our life together. That isn't necessary. Yet perhaps I should refer, although briefly, to Eusebio's rather remarkable professional career — also forgotten.

A few years after our wedding and after the birth of our children, Eloísa and Jaime, we moved from Madrid to Cáceres where he worked as a journalist on a regional newspaper. Cáceres is in the Spanish province of Extremadura, which shares a boundary with Portugal in the west, Salamanca in the north and Andalucía in the south. It is a quaint city of some one hundred thousand souls today, although when we were there in the 1970s, the population barely reached sixty thousand. It can boast, however, of having one of the most beautiful historical quarters in Spain. That was where he also found his niche — in politics. With his sharp, critical mind, he upset the somewhat stale management of the newspaper when he would criticise some of the decisions taken by certain provincial authorities. We all know that in small towns anybody who boasts of being *someone* is known by everyone. This means that criticism is doubly painful because it is aired in bars and restaurants and soon the amiable Director of the *Diario de Extremadura* could no longer bear the accusations of tolerating that rebellious columnist on his staff! He reacted by taking Eusebio's column, *El Polvo de los Días*, out of the paper and relegating him to correcting proofs. For a free spirit that was the end of his journalistic career and it was when he began to get involved in politics.

He had always been concerned about the future of his people after the long years of Franco's dictatorship and to add his grain of sand to Spain's incipient democracy was a logical step for him. During those eight years in Cáceres, he became General Secretary of the Socialist Party there and also MP for Cáceres in Spain's National Parliament, *Las Cortes*. I think I am right in saying that he really preferred those years in the provinces, where he spent the early hours of the morning debating strategies with his bearded revolutionary friends around ashtrays full of cigarette butts, to the cold, carpeted corridors of the Spanish Parliament in the more staid Madrid. Eusebio had always been a genuine, sincere person and he found his work in Cáceres more useful than being a mere cog in the wheel of national politics. That said, we both tired of provincial life and, as he had to spend several days each week in Parliament in Madrid, we decided to move back there. We risked changing the religious schools of Eloísa and Jaime for a State school in Madrid. That wasn't easy for them but, little by little, all of us managed to feel happier in the large metropolis.

However, that was not the final step in Eusebio's profession. Several years later he was elected as Spanish MP for Cáceres to the European Parliament in Brussels. It was an opportunity for him — the apex of his career — and also for us. Elo and Jaime could attend the European School, an enormous establishment with none less than three thousand pupils divided into some eight different linguistic sections, a true Tower of Babel. And we remained there during two political terms, eight years. It was a good experience, yet all four of us missed Spain and Eusebio, in particular, tired of his constant journeys to far-flung lands in the company of people in whom he had little interest, of his parliamentary debates amidst those who often turned a deaf ear, of his distancing from the national politics of his homeland, which had initially so enthused him back in Cáceres. And, above all, it was time for a new challenge — he was thinking about renovating the small house we had bought a few years previously in Madrid, renovating it with his own hands. And with ours! Two years of cement, bricks, iron beams, iron bars on the windows, paint and the embellishment of floors and walls. Some workmen helped us, obviously, but we did a great deal with our own efforts. Another unforgettable experience. Some say that when a couple builds a house, they are cemented together for life! Yet that too, he forgot.

Once the house was finished, he began to write. Another challenge. He wrote several novels, managing to publish three of them, others were relegated to the drawers of his study. When he realised that they had received only scant public notice, he gave up on his literary efforts and dedicated his time to more artistic pursuits, making decorative objects and painting them for the garden and the house. At that time he read for hours and we also went a great deal to the cinema, to the theatre and to concerts. But, gradually, he left off everything, his interest waned for anything outside himself and his immediate needs.

Our Enemy

It is difficult, almost impossible, to know with exactitude when his illness began, when his forgetfulness, when his life — and indeed ours beside him — started to alter. I do know that his first visit to a neurologist was back in 2014, six years ago now. And why did we take him to the neurologist? Simply because we began to notice failings in his memory and proof of that was the record he had always made of our banking movements. He had always kept a meticulous account of our spending and our income. But I began to notice that he no longer seemed to know what amounts coincided with the different concepts and, instead of making a correct note of the pensions we receive, he would write down anything at all in an unintelligible scribble.

Then it hit me that he had nothing but confusion in his mind. A little later we had some workmen in the house and we had to pay them. He went off to the bank with a cheque in his pocket for the exaggerated amount of seven thousand euros. Fortunately, it happened to be a public holiday and the bank was closed, but he could so easily have lost the cheque made out to the bearer. I took it away from him. The following day, which was Saturday, he repeated his action with another cheque, this time to the sum of five thousand euros, also made out to the bearer! That was more than a warning.

Throughout all our married days we had never been accustomed to going together as a couple to the doctor or dentist. Many couples always accompany each other on those occasions, but we maintained a certain independence of movement which meant that we often didn't coincide over appointments for one thing or the other. So, when he would return from a visit to the clinic and I would ask him what the results of his analysis had been, he would simply reply "nothing". And the same thing happened when he went out to lunch with friends. When he returned home I would ask him about his outing and he would just say "nothing". That reply began to concern me. Did he really have no interest in his friends, or was it that he couldn't remember what they had talked about?

One of our neighbours, a DIY handyman just like Eusebio, also from León, told me that he too was worried about him because, when he came over to help him out in the garden, he realised that Eusebio couldn't remember what it was he had to do, which tools he had to look for; in short, he was mixing things up. Then, almost immediately afterwards, he didn't remember what they had been doing together. This man's mother had died of Alzheimer's. He and his partner had cared for her and so, fortunately for me, he was aware of the implications of the illness.

This was when I noticed that Eusebio's enthusiasm for certain tasks began to wane and his habits changed. There are several examples of this.

We have a Norwegian wood stove, admired by all and which provided so much warmth, both physical and spiritual, inside our home, in particular in the lounge area. It also heated other nearby areas of the house and I can remember that we used to love sitting beside it, gazing into its flames as they danced in tune to our thoughts, enchanted by its orange-yellow colours, staring fixedly at it into the early hours of the morning as the flames subsided turning into golden embers and then into ash. A wood fire induces dreams. It was as though we were in a little village as the smell from our chimney reached the neighbours' houses and flats, but they never complained about that. On the contrary, they seemed to enjoy it.

My duties with the stove were to clean out the ash every morning, taking it out to the earth in the garden to serve as fertiliser for the plants, to sweep out the inside of the stove and to clean the glass windows which were blackened daily by the smoke. Eusebio's job was to feed it with large logs of wood. Each year we ordered four or five thousand kilos of seasoned oak. He used to have to go outside four or five times a day to bring in the logs that we kept underneath the stairway at the entrance to the garden, not always such a pleasant journey if it was particularly cold or happened to be raining or snowing. The stove was greedy and had to be fed almost incessantly. Yet one day he tired of bringing in the wood and lighting the fire (as a city girl, I was always disastrous with that, finding it hard to make the wood catch light). He tired too of staring into the flames of the stove and it was as though he had forgotten that it had symbolised something beloved and essential to his well-being. As it had done for me. Our daughter Eloísa, for her part, detested the smell in our lounge, the smell of fire and wood that other people liked she found suffocating and a health threat. I also tired of cleaning it out daily and I certainly appreciated not having to spend my days feeding it with logs. And so it is several years now that the stove has stood there clean and empty, a decorative piece more than anything else and Eusebio never even referred to it after that. Now we heat our radiators with a gas-fired boiler; it is cleaner and easier. And so it is that my companion began to lose interest in the things he had always loved in life, and gradually began to change.

* * *

There were other signs. I recall moments which were exceedingly embarrassing when he would burst into fits of temper with others in the family, with friends, with people on the metro or in the cinema if they happened to be blocking the exit. Once he simply couldn't wait at the end of a film when they were showing the interminable list of credits and music in the darkness. He felt an obsessive need to leave the cinema as soon as the film was over. All I could do was to follow. And this happened a lot. I disliked having to pick my way down the steps that I couldn't see.

"Why all this hurry?" I once asked. But the man was impatient and on that particular occasion, he leapt from his seat in a fury flinging abuses to all and sundry and almost falling over the poor woman beside me who was lame and was blocking the way with her two crutches. His outbursts were out of all proportion. Eusebio had always, throughout his whole life, had a quick temper which he often found hard to control. Instead of stopping, putting the event into proportion, he would lose his calm and shout abusively beyond all measure. Psychologists might say that he was furious because of his own shortcomings. That happens. Sometimes all of us tend to blame someone else if we feel trapped. And he would do this quite often. I must admit it was a negative side to his character for those of us who lived with him. It seemed that we no longer lived with him. However, it was that same temperament which was at the source of many of his successes in life and which had prevented him from collapsing under difficulties. It guaranteed him success in his profession and in many things that others would have deemed impossible. He was tenacious and exceptionally patient when concluding any task that he had set his heart on, yet he was not so patient with others.

I felt saddened at those outbursts of anger when he used to argue over the phone with his political friends, literally telling them to get lost if they didn't agree with him. We lost friendships with people we had known during his time in the European Parliament. Little by little they stopped phoning and he was incapable of making peace with them, or of recognising that he'd overstepped the mark. I can also remember several very complicated situations with people he would insult on the metro because, immersed as they were in their conversations, they wouldn't get out of the way when we had to get out of the train. I was almost scared to go on the metro with him and I used to tell him to be more careful; someone might return his insult or do something even worse. There was a long period of time when he used to behave really badly with one of our best friends, insulting her with ugly words every time he saw her. She put up with him stoically and thankfully that period hasn't affected our friendship. After that, the problem seemed to be her husband, and when we went out for lunch we had to separate the two men.

I have read that Cézanne, the post-Impressionist artist, used to delight in being uncouth when he was in "exquisite" company; it is said that the more elegant the Parisian salons where he was exhibiting his works of art, the more unfriendly and unsociable he became. He was a solitary soul, even amongst his contemporaries. Eusebio had something of this about him, although he had always been very shy in social circles when outside his own comfort zone, for example, in the European Parliament in the midst of a multitude of foreign tongues. He never even managed to speak good English despite all our years together. I was a bad teacher, he always said. Maybe. But he never showed the slightest interest in learning English. The French he had learnt in the seminary of his youth, in Paris and later in Brussels, was enough for him. But he was never happy trying to express himself in a language other than his native Spanish. As to his social shyness and his impatience, I tend to blame his infancy for that facet of his personality, a childhood of unjust punishments in freezing cold seminaries in the icy winters of rural León. In those days, the Catholic Church was partly responsible for moulding its pupils, preparing them for a life of abnegation, filled with guilt and loathing for all aspects of terrestrial life. They were many, those formative years lived in the solitude and stringency of the monastic life. It was bound to affect Eusebio throughout all his days, as indeed it did with several of his friends who had experienced that same upbringing. That was why he always hated the church which, despite himself, lay within the very marrow of his bones.

* * *

I have much time alone. Time to reflect. If I go backwards in time, back in search of some of the beginnings of my companion's illness, I can recall the hours and hours when he would sit outside in his garden in the sun during the long afternoons of the Madrid summer, those hours when the world seems to be asleep. Indeed, it was siesta time. He would also sleep, yet most of the time he would sit, barely moving, without reacting to our comments except for an almost imperceptible movement of his head, or he would raise his arm, but rarely would he bother to get involved in an answer to any question.

During those prolonged silences, was he thinking, was he remembering his life, was he dreaming, or was he simply in harmony with his surroundings, with the song of the birds, the movement of the leaves in a light breeze, with the voices from the street, the passing cars? For a long time he seemed to be obsessed by the voice of one of our neighbours and I believe that he used to dream of intimacies with her. It seems that this is very common in older men, that desire for new flesh, for extra-marital experiences. It is normal. It is life, I suppose. One doesn't have to feel humiliated or be angry over it. At the end of the day, each to his own desires. As life shortens and, with it, sexual desire, dreams of unattainable things become more intense. Dreams are all that is left.

He no longer read nor wrote. Yet he had read and written so much, as a journalist and politician. After having published, as I have already said, three novels with little success and having sent his work to numerous editors who refused it, I believe that he lost interest in trying to publish.

He never wrote for the pleasure of the activity in itself, he wrote for an audience and he would say: "Why go on writing if nobody reads it?" He wrote extremely well. He had always loved good literature and he chose his words and phrases with subtlety and elegance. But was that enough to please a reader? He often wrote bitterly, issuing truths like meting out blows. He wasn't interested in nice little stories, in love stories or in adventure stories. He wrote about life, about his childhood village, about the death of his mother, about those terrible years in the seminary, about experiences he had lived and which were familiar to him. He rarely made novels out of his thoughts.

I consider that the result of his creative efforts was excellent, both for the content and for the way he expressed himself. He had a fine sense of observation and never beat about the bush. Yet above all he was literary, a writer who respected his language and who used it in a beautiful way and with exceptional sensitivity. It is sad that he never achieved the success he sought. Had he done so, I am convinced that he would have continued writing. And he would have continued reading.

True, even before, he didn't read compulsively every day, not even every week, but when he picked up a book he wouldn't put it down until he had finished it. And yes, he read a lot. Perhaps, however, the fact that he no longer read and no longer wrote didn't have so much to do with his lack of success as a writer. Perhaps it was more the illness that was quietly nibbling at the neurones and synapses in his brain, preventing him from remembering a page read, preventing him from having the necessary concentration to put his thoughts into words.

Throughout his adult life Eusebio had always enjoyed driving. When we lived in Cáceres he would drive for hours and hours visiting villages during the electoral campaigns. He had always enjoyed travelling. We used to make a lot of journeys all over Spain. Holidays in the north, in Galicia, Asturias, Santander, the Picos de Europa (the continuation of the Pyrenees Mountains towards the west passing through the provinces of Santander, León and Asturias) and the Basque Country, another year in Catalonia, Girona, the Costa Brava, also further down the coast in Valencia and Alicante, the coastline of Cádiz in the far south, all the provinces of Andalusia passing through La Mancha and, of course, Castilla-León, then another year in Lisbon driving right through Portugal from south to north.

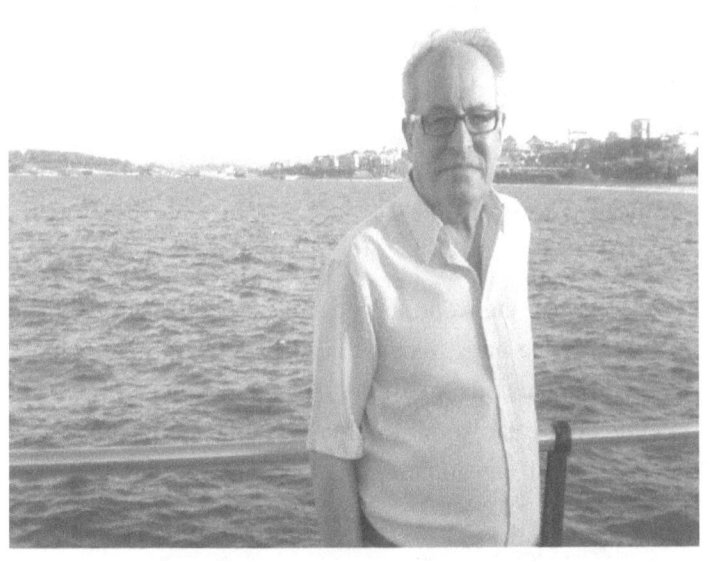

Santander Bay, September 2014

We gobbled up kilometres, always avid to discover new places, historical buildings, panoramic views. Not to forget those lengthy journeys that we did on many an occasion between Madrid and Brussels whilst we lived up there, passing through Paris. We used to share the wheel of the car, but Eusebio loved driving and could go on for hours without stopping. Yet very gradually I began to realise that he couldn't remember routes that should have been familiar to him and he would ask me more and more where he had to turn off a road. He was losing control and the best thing was for him not to drive any more. Did he miss it? He never even referred to it, not a word, not even one evening when I insisted on driving him from Eloísa's house to ours. He never asked about the car which we left to our son Jaime because he is the one who needs it. In Madrid, the public transport was more than sufficient for us or perhaps a taxi if we needed to go to the hospital and Eusebio was feeling weak.

But like the wood for the stove, like his control of the money and the bank, like calling in workmen, or attending to any bureaucratic questions, like his own writing and reading, the car also slid out of his life as though it had never been of any importance. So many things forgotten now forever.

* * *

For a long time, when I realised that my companion seemed to be losing the ability to concentrate, I suggested we play chess, dominos, Scrabble, in the evenings, anything which would have meant he had to use his mind. I thought it would help. On the first visit we made to the neurologist, Eusebio was given some books full of exercises to stimulate the mind. There was no way that I could make him participate in any of those activities. He shunned them off as stupidities for children, for idiots, but the truth was that he was incapable of following them himself. Quickly I saw that I could never draw him out of his lethargy in that way. And so we spent our evenings in front of the television. For me it was an escape and often really interesting. But for him it wasn't any more than a confusing mixture of images that he couldn't understand or analyse or even remember the next morning. For me, to a certain extent, it replaced the cinema where we often used to go once or twice a week, always to good films that he also enjoyed watching. But soon I realised that what he was seeing meant nothing at all to him. He would start to whistle, utterly withdrawn into himself and oblivious to the film or to those around him. It was the same when we used to go to concerts, especially those given by young pianists and so obviously we couldn't continue going to those. He wouldn't stop whistling and that annoys people, particularly if they are trying to listen to music! But it was a loss only to me.

The whistling was also annoying in the waiting room of a hospital, or on a train or bus. I recall a journey by train that we made to Cádiz when two passengers complained, asking him to stop whistling, and on another occasion the driver of the coach coming back from Granada, where we had spent several days with close friends, also asked him to stop. That was the time we journeyed with friends for miles by car, going from one white town in Andalusia to another. It was a fascinating trip with olive groves on each side of the road, climbing high between biblical rocks, drinking in vast and magnificent views and visiting historical buildings. Eusebio sat whistling in the back of the car, constantly asking our friends where they were taking us. On public transport, although I tried desperately hard to stop him, he would keep on and on whistling the same tune over and over again in his own little isolated world and I would have to apologise to the other passengers.

All this made me realise that little by little we would have to give up doing more and more things. I also realised that anyway, he wasn't getting anything at all out of going here, there and everywhere. He was never a particularly sociable person; he never felt the need to search for company in clubs or associations or reading or culture circles. He was quite happy to sit tranquilly in his garden, in the garden where he had worked like a native, listening to the birds, watching the leaves of the nineteen trees he had planted, feeling the embrace of the sunlight and its warmth on his skin. And so we had to reduce our outings considerably. One adapts. You don't gain anything protesting against what life has in store for you at this stage. We had seen a great deal. We had travelled a lot. We'd had a better life than we could ever have dreamt of. So why complain?

Eusebio was always a very practical person, incredibly logical and often incapable of understanding that people and life are not always rational. However, his pragmatism also suffered. He simply couldn't enter into the recycling era. As I wanted him to help me and to do something instead of doing nothing at all, I used to ask him to take the rubbish bins out. He could never understand that the plastics and cartons had to go into the yellow bin, other rubbish into the grey bin with an orange lid and, lastly, the remains of food into the bin with a brown lid. I would see him from the window of my study go out into the garden and, instead of putting the bags in the assigned bin, what he used to do was to take all the bags containing plastics and place them in the grey bin for other rubbish! Then he would leave it outside to be collected. It was useless trying to explain to him the idea of putting each bag in its proper place, quite impossible. The more I tried to explain it to him, the more confused he seemed. Then, even more disheartening, the following morning, he would bring some other neighbour's bin in from the street instead of ours. Could it all be so difficult?

I realise that recycling is a relatively new concept, with the importance of being able to recycle certain objects harmful to the environment having now been recognized, batteries, electronic apparatus, paper, bottles, etc. And we are now able to use the remains of food, of which there are large amounts in our society of plenty, with those remains going to compost that can then be converted into biomass destined for providing energy. Ten years ago all this was inconceivable. Nobody worried about it until we became aware of the tremendous harm we are doing to our oceans, our environment, to the entire planet, amassing millions and millions of tons of all sorts of rubbish. But all this came late in life to my companion. He no longer had the neurons to be able to cope with these matters. He wasn't capable of learning new things. He had enough with what was left of what he had known all his life and even that had long since floated out of his head.

Thinking that I was making the kitchen safer for him, we installed a new induction plate in the kitchen for cooking, with controls where you have to slide your finger to left or right for the required degree of heat. It's difficult to hurt yourself because the plaque turns itself off once you take the saucepan away and if you forget to turn off the hobs then they switch off automatically a minute later. But if you put your fingers on one of them straight after withdrawing the saucepan, when it is still hot, even though there is no flame and it isn't red, then you might burn yourself. However, the day after it was installed, Eusebio stared at it intensely asking where the flame and the gas was. I tried to teach him to use the controls, but that was too much for him and he never ever tried to heat even his own tea for breakfast, whereas he could do that with gas. Ironically, all we had done was to make him more dependent on others.

Another innovation in the house which we thought would improve our quality of life given his increasing incapacity is the automatic answering machine, or intercom, which has a small screen in the lounge so you can see who is at the gate. It is extremely practical particularly as there is quite a way from the house to the front gate and when you see who it is, then you can open the gate by pressing a button inside the house. On the other hand, if you see that there is some undesirable character whom you don't want to let in, then you don't have to open. It is a wonderful system especially for older people, very easy and, particularly, during these years when we have less energy to go outside to answer the door when someone calls. Yet all that happened was that Eusebio was confused by the little red light that shines constantly on the apparatus on the lounge wall. Almost every single night he would ask: What is that light? I also tried to explain how to open the door with the button, but every time someone rang the doorbell, he would call me to open the door, or confuse it with the telephone. There are four buttons on the video panel; all with different functions, which is enough to confound any normal mind, but for him it was impossible and perhaps, too, that was preferable because he didn't have sufficient judgement to decide who could or could not come in. It was the sad reality, yet fortunately he seemed to accept without question that there were certain things he could no longer do.

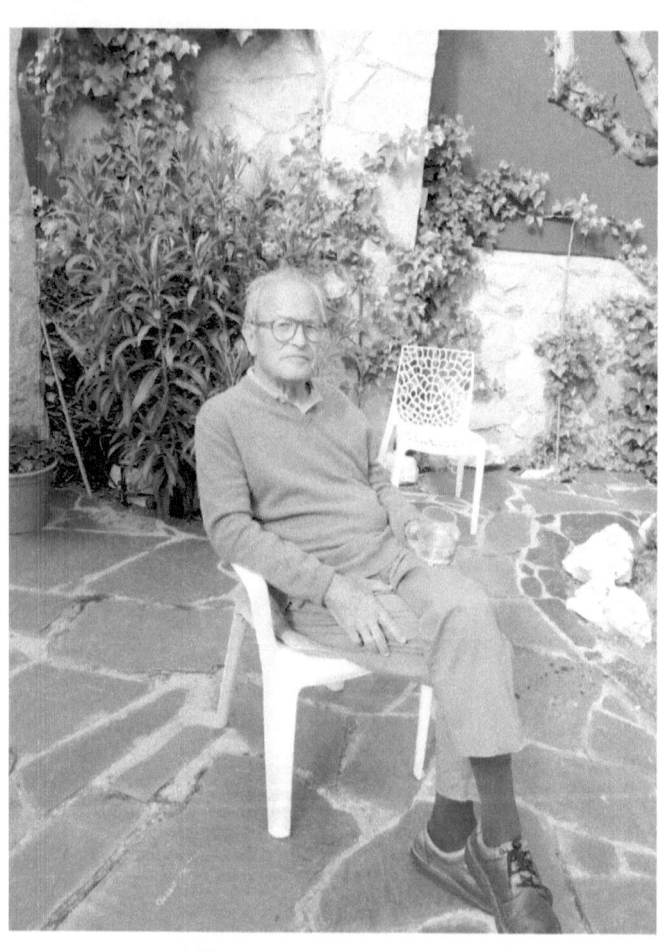
Whiling away the hours in his garden

An Escapade

A short time after the intercom was installed, Eusebio treated us to a more dramatic adventure. I realise that Alzheimer patients tend to get disoriented and there are lots of cases where they go outside the house or residence where they live and they get irremediably lost because they very often don't even recognise the street where their home is or the surroundings of their own district, or the places they have seen a thousand times on walks. They leave the house and go off a long way from their starting point, wandering along in response to some impulse in their brain which impels them to go on this adventure. I don't believe that it is a conscious desire to escape from home, certainly not. It is simply another confused element in their days full of confusion.

I used to allow my companion to go out alone because I wanted him to have a little independence and because I knew that he never went very far and, also, the people in the district knew him. Eusebio was always a man of set ways and he never used to go further than Arturo Soria, two minutes from home where he used to sit on one of the wooden benches and spend his time watching the passers-by, old people, young people, young men and, in particular, young women, as they walked along the pavement. He would go out after his siesta and go straight to his bench in Arturo Soria for a couple of hours, no more.

A couple of hours which that day, at the end of September, turned into over ten!

I recall that before going out that afternoon he had awoken from his siesta confused. He asked me where he had to go. I responded that he didn't have to go anywhere, just to Arturo Soria to his bench as he always did. He went off and then, after he hadn't returned, the young son of one of our neighbours, told me that about five o'clock when he had come home from school, he had seen Eusebio walking up and down the street beside the house seemingly very confused. At seven thirty, when he still hadn't returned, I started to worry. I went out to look for him. He wasn't on "his bench". I couldn't see him in the street. I asked at the chemist, in the shops of a nearby road, and in the baker's but nobody had seen him go by the whole afternoon. As soon as I returned home I called the police, giving them a description of him and how he was dressed, in short sleeves because it was still hot during the afternoon although the nights were cooler. I called my children and, with our hearts in our mouths, we began the search, together with our neighbours Susana, Mar and José Luis. It is marvellous how friends respond in times of need.

The worst thing at such times is the anxiety of the unknown. Where was he, what was he doing, was he completely lost, had some undesirable person hurt him, had he fallen and hurt himself? Our son Jaime took the car down one side of Arturo Soria which is a street over six kilometres long and its adjoining streets while Juan, Elo's partner, drove down the other side. Eloísa went to the police to formally lodge a missing person's notice, which took her about two hours because of the long queue there. I felt totally useless staying at home, even though we knew that someone had to be there in case Eusebio turned up at the door. And what if he had lost his keys? He had never used a mobile phone, or a computer. This world of modern technology had completely by-passed him. He couldn't even turn on the television as it is now by cable. He absolutely refused one day when I attempted to teach him how to use the computer just for writing and, since then, he never wanted to know about it anymore. He would never even take any proof of identity in his pockets and all he had was a chain round his neck with his name and our phone numbers engraved on it. I gave him that chain for his birthday doubting that he would wear it, but when I told him it was a medal for having reached seventy-seven years, he never took it off. It wasn't very obvious as identification, but perhaps better than nothing.

Finally, at about one o'clock in the morning Elo, Jaime and Juan returned to the house exhausted, their faces fraught with concern. He wasn't to be found anywhere. We were absolutely desperate, the hours passed so slowly. We didn't want to say anything to the rest of the family so as not to alarm them. If he didn't turn up by the next morning, then we would have to tell them. What could they possibly do in the middle of the night? The police were looking for him and would tell us if they found him. But the hours passed and the police didn't call. I couldn't resist ringing them a couple of times to ask, but they said they were searching for all they were worth and it was preferable if I didn't call again because it was more of a nuisance to them than anything else. So we had no option but to wait! Oh Lord! We were all on the point of exploding, worrying and imagining him in the worst possible situations, perhaps he had dirtied himself because, since his colon cancer operation, he used to wear a colostomy bag. We imagined him in pain, unable to call for help, lost in a deserted street somewhere in the city. The police had asked us where he used to work because these patients often return to places of the past, even to where they had been brought up. Could he have tried to go off to León, 350 kms away? Had some driver picked him up seeing him wandering along the side of the motorway? We had called the local bars, the petrol station shop where he used to go daily for the newspaper, and also his Day Centre. Nothing. No-one had seen him.

The truth is that all those hours of waiting had left us with an enormous emptiness in our stomachs, terror in our hearts and such an intense emotion that it was impossible to think with any clarity. Finally, at three-thirty in the morning, ten and a half hours after he had left home, the telephone rang. It was the police. But not the police from Chamartín or Canillas districts, close to home. It was the police from Alcorcón, no less than thirty-five kilometres outside Madrid! Eusebio was there in the police station with them and they told us to come immediately to pick him up. The four of us left in Juan's car, discussing during the whole three-quarter-of-an-hour journey how he had ended up there. We imagined that someone had taken him in a car, but why, we didn't know. How on earth could he have ended up so far from home? We considered that perhaps he had got onto the Extremadura road, where we went so often when we lived in Cáceres and that someone had seen him wandering along the side of the motorway. So many things cross the mind at times like that, a mixed sea of phantoms.

When we arrived at the police station in Alcorcón, with the help of Juan's GPS, we saw him absolutely alone, except for a receptionist, sitting on one of the benches in the hall, whistling no less, perfectly happy in the silence around him. When we went up to him, full of relief with smiles all over our faces, he looked at us and asked, "What on earth are you doing here?" As calm as the night outside, would you believe it! As though nothing had happened. He had no idea how he had got there, nor why he was there, nor where he actually was, nor where he had been. The happiness of the innocent! He only had four metro maps in his pocket and had spent the few euros he had. The police told us that he had arrived at the metro station Parque de Lisboa late at night and that the guard in the metro, realising he was confused and understanding that he was searching for a hospital which didn't exist there, called the Police immediately. He had left home with barely four or five euros in his pocket and didn't have a metro pass. We couldn't imagine how he had gone so far. He must have been hours and hours going round in circles in the metro, changing trains at one station or another. I imagined that he must have felt so much anxiety. However, none of that showed on his face, only calm and stability. He wasn't hungry, thirsty, he wasn't frightened, or lonely, or cold. It was as though nothing at all had happened to him. On the contrary, he appeared to have had a good time! Nothing like what he had made us go through.

It is precisely that lack of consciousness which helps Alzheimer patients to suffer their condition with equanimity, at least during certain stages of the illness. They don't seem to feel cold, or heat, or hunger, or frustration, they don't recognise dishes of food that they liked or did not like, they don't remember if they have had breakfast or not, if they have taken coffee after their meal, if they have had supper or not. They don't worry about anything at all and with no preoccupations, with no unpleasant memories, with no awareness of what is going on in the world, the wrinkles fall from their faces.

And the Days Go By

At that time, Eusebio expressed everything by whistling. He whistled for hours a day, he incessantly whistled the same song that none of us recognised, although our niece Silvia, said she thought she did, a song recuperated from some hidden cranny of his village youth or when he was in the seminary where he spent so many years, some twelve in all until he was able to free himself from that persecuted existence when he was twenty-one or twenty-two. That constant whistling could be a tremendous nuisance to the person at his side, who was generally me, because it interrupts your concentration over the book you are reading, the TV programme which interests you, or it simply disturbs your own thoughts. However, that said, I should say that whistling was far better than any screams or outbursts of bad temper. I even thought that as he was incapable of participating in a conversation, it was his way of affirming himself in life, his way of telling us that he was still alive and kicking, that he should be taken into account and that he was certainly not at his end, despite his memory failure. But maybe that's just me trying to give meaning to the meaningless.

Almost two years ago now, Catón, one of our beautiful cats died. He was an imposing male with a strong character, yet also with a tenderness not common in cats. He was sure of himself and of his place in the family beside his sister Alba. He was a dominating cat and seemingly strong. Yet on the sad afternoon of Sunday, December 2, 2018, he collapsed in the kitchen. He vomited and we took him to an emergency vet. She did all she could to save his life, his lungs were congested and his heart had failed him. Eloisa, Juan, Eusebio and I went to say goodbye to him as she gave him the injection to put him to sleep. It was a terribly sad moment because he was a cat with a marvellous personality.

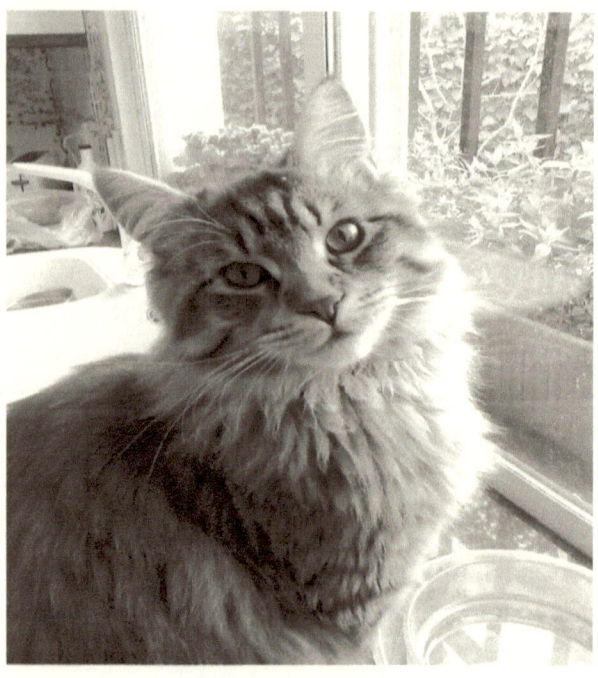

Catón, our beautiful cat, now deceased

Eusebio had no recollection at all of that moment, nor of the cat himself, but I am not exaggerating when I say that he spent months after Caton´s death asking at least five times every night where the *other cat* was. "He isn't here anymore", I would say, "he died, he is dead". Dead? he repeated. Then he would ask me again half an hour later, or less. He didn't seem to miss him, neither did he remember him at all during the day or if I showed him a photo of the animal, but it was obvious that when night fell and we locked ourselves in the lounge, with our other cat, Alba, it was then that he missed the other presence. He showed no sadness for the cat's death. He repeated, absolutely cold — "dead!" — without any sentiment at all, simply affirming an evident truth.

It made me sadder than him. Losing an animal who has been a pet for years is exceptionally hard. Losing a loved one is more than exceptionally hard, yet there is something about the defencelessness of an animal which needles its way into our souls. The company an animal gives to man, that unconditional love and admiration and affection, their dependence on you, makes the relationship very special. And, of course, an animal never answers you back!

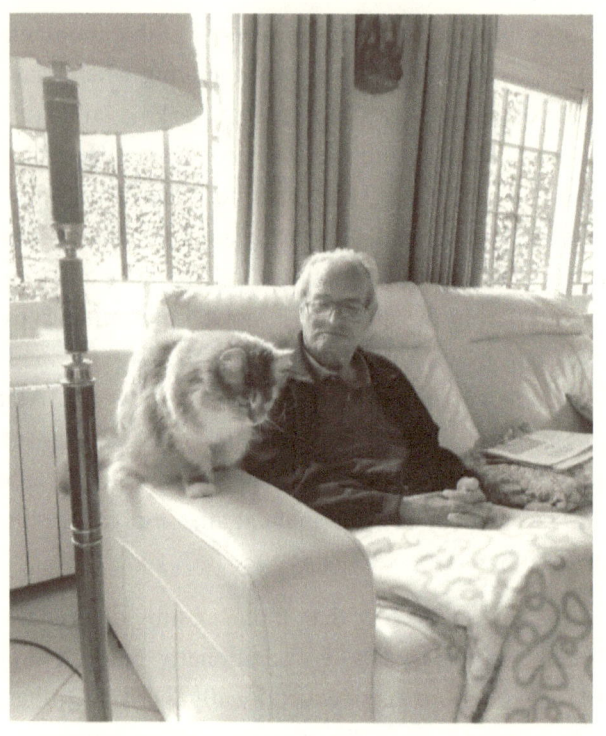

On the lounge sofa beside Alba, February 2020

Eusebio used to get up late every morning. After all, what did he have to do? The day no longer beckoned him with seductive or interesting activities. He was a man who had lost his sense of direction and smell and taste, physically and not only intellectually, whose hearing was going, he hadn't heard well for a long time and he never wished to remedy that by wearing a hearing aid. Therefore he auto-excluded himself from being able to participate actively in our reunions with family and friends. When we still communicated, we used to say to him: "But you wear glasses for your sight, why not wear a hearing aid?" No way! He was obstinate about it without giving us a convincing answer. Was he scared, perhaps, of not being able to control the apparatus? Who knows? He no longer enjoyed reading. He had lost interest in books a long time back. What a pity, especially for the aged, because reading enriches the hours which go more slowly in old age, when one loses interest in doing so many things in the world outside. The time flies more and more with advancing years, but the hours go slowly. He had completely changed. The newspaper and the news no longer interested him either. He had forgotten those who were to the forefront of politics in our time, people he used to like or who irritated him for what he considered the wrong decisions they took. He forgot the people in his political party, the PSOE, where he had dedicated so many years of his life with enthusiasm and where he had developed his love for politics at a time which was particularly interesting, even passionate, in Spain, the transition from the fascist Franco era to democracy. He no longer even knew who was the top man in the party. If the neurologists asked him who the Prime Minister was, he would reply, after a long pause, Felipe González. That was a long time ago! Since then, everything had fled from his brain.

Neither did he want to get up to go outside into his garden where previously, he used to spend hours and hours caring for his plants, his trees, sweeping up the autumn leaves, pruning the roses at the end of winter. He didn't stop and would happily spend whole mornings occupied outside, content in his solitary work. He had green fingers, as the English say about people who make plants grow well and who love them. He used to enjoy going to the nursery to choose flowers, seeds, bushes, vines, anything to beautify the garden. I recall two journeys we made to Valencia, for no less a reason than to buy a mandarin tree. So endearing and pretty. I came with it in the back of the car with the seats collapsed, each and every one of the 350 kms from Valencia, hugging its small, robust trunk. We were so excited with our purchase. We planted it and Eusebio constructed a sort of umbrella to protect it from the icy mornings in winter. It lasted two years, but then its leaves began to fall, it became sadder each day, nostalgic for the salty air of its Valencian orchard. But we didn't give up.

The second journey to Valencia was this time to buy an orange tree and that little tree with its two juicy oranges arrived on a lorry with the proprietor of the nursery. He was animated and sure it would flourish here. Alas! It didn't. The following winter it also began to wilt and so the day came when we had to take it out of the earth with its drooping branches and sapless trunk. We then realised that it was preferable to plant only bushes which were suited to Madrid. We also gave a turn to two Australian bushes, the grevillea with its delicate, spider-like flowers and soft wavy leaves; and a bottle brush, that tree with a red flower in the shape of a round oblong brush. They ended up like the citrus trees. And two bright pink bougainvilleas went the same way. There are simply specimens of nature which ought to stay in their original surroundings and all of the ones I have mentioned come from the coast where they flourish in the salty air which blows in from the sea. Madrid is a long way from the sea.

But why should he have bothered to get out of bed, now that all that activity had died for him? He saw no sense in absolutely anything outside, nor perhaps in anything at all, except to sit for hours in the sun immersed in his own thoughts, or immersed in the confusion or the void that had assailed his brain and which perhaps for brief moments, only for brief moments, steeped him in profound sadness.

What he did do then was to water the garden, but not with the hose. For quite some time I could see him from the window of my study searching for a corner outside to urinate. I don't know if this was because of some sort of ancestral pleasure, taking into account that when we married, as I mentioned, there was no running water in the village home, so throughout his youth he had had to go outside to satisfy nature's call. It was a normal thing then and, of course, in the countryside it is not a problem. Yet ever since we have known each other we have always had access to a bathroom, except in those very early years when in the village. It was only very recently that I would see him using the earth round one of the trees. And I didn't mind. What I did mind was when he awoke from his siesta, often confused, and would go off looking for the toilet if the weather was bad outside and then he would find it in my study, or in the piano room or in the dining area, or in the hall. It must have been the urgency of the moment that disoriented him and I was not always aware of what he was doing. That was for number one. For number two, and I suppose that was somewhat of a relief, he had worn a colostomy bag since his operation for colon cancer in the autumn of 2017. Unfortunately, he was incapable of understanding what happened in that bag, except if he was in the nude and could see the matter coming out uncontrollably. But he was never able to change the bag or to clean himself. Frankly it was a most unpleasant task for me as I am not a nurse or a professional carer. But it is incredible the things one accepts out of duty and love for a patient. Also because there was no alternative. I mean, what could I have done? Have had a nurse available in the house day and night just in case the wretched bag had to be changed? No. One did it, and that was that. But I am no martyr and I have to admit that it was one of the tasks that I would happily have put aside if I could have done so.

Eating was less of an issue. His mental confusion led him on occasions to pick at the cat's food. I put it on the kitchen bench surface in the morning and would leave it for a few hours before washing the dish. If Eusebio went into the kitchen before lunch because he was obviously hungry and liked to nibble, he would go straight to the cat's bowl.

Animal food is neither tasty nor pleasant to our palate, but he didn't realise. It must have seemed to him like nuts or almonds. But at least this wasn't a daily habit with him.

Another problem he had was with dressing. It became more and more difficult for him. As I wanted him to continue doing as much as he could by himself, I used to place his toothbrush with the toothpaste, his soap, his brush and razor for shaving, his comb, all these things placed beside the bathroom washbasin, his towel too and his clothing visibly hung up where he could see it. Even then, he made mistakes. I remember the day when I went to see if I could help him to dress and I found him sitting on the side of the bed wearing a pair of woollen leggings. I wondered where he had found them because neither of us had leggings like that. On closer inspection I realised that he had put his legs into the armholes of one of his woollen jackets. I almost cried, his incapacity was so sad. There were times when he forgot to take off his pyjamas or he put his vest on top of his jersey, or his winter shoes without socks. And one night he got undressed and I found him literally imprisoned with his arms in a piece of clothing, fighting to free himself. He had forced his head and arms into the pyjama shorts which were his summer pyjamas. He had become completely unable to carry out any task at all, however easy. Yes, he still shaved himself alone on most mornings, but worse and worse. And when he showered I had to be there with him constantly, otherwise he would mix the body gel with the hair shampoo.

His confusion also affected his words, well, the few words he then uttered. He mixed up the names of objects. Normally it was fairly easy for me to know what he meant when he put his hands into his pockets and asked me where his 'scissors' were, where is my 'load', he would say. Before he escaped to Alcorcón, he used to have keys, a handkerchief and a little money, just a few coins. I let him have this so that he felt he had money of his own and also because, for years and years, he used to go to the bread shop to buy our daily bread. I wanted him, as I have already said, to feel useful in some way. Buying the bread and the paper was his daily duty. In fact, he had done this for the last fifty years almost every single day. That gave him an opportunity to walk a little as well. And so, yes, he had his 'load' in his trouser pocket.

However, after Alcorcón, I took all the money away from him and, obviously, the house keys - Twice you've lost them, I said to him and I had to call in the locksmith to change the lock on the gate as I didn't want to risk anyone coming into the house. He seemed to understand. Sometimes he would go up the stairs to the gate and try to open the lock, but realised that he couldn't and so he would come down into the kitchen for a knife. Then he would go up again. That didn't work. He came down again and went to his shed where he kept his tools and went up the stairs again, this time with a screwdriver. No luck. Four or five times he went up and down the steps to the gate, but came down again without protesting or saying anything at all. In fact, I really think that by the time he had come down the steps he had forgotten why he had gone up them. And so his keys became 'scissors'. He even called lunch the 'record'. When are we going to have the 'record'? "Where are my 'pippets'?" he asked, staring at the coffee table in the lounge, because he had forgotten to put his glasses on during those days when he didn't want to dress and would stay in pyjamas all day long. That didn't happen often but, yes, very occasionally. And once when the lounge was being painted they had dismounted everything and he said, "but where are the 'hotels'," indicating the walls with a vague gesture. "Ah, you mean the paintings?" I answered him.

I believe that it is fairly frequent in Alzheimer patients for them to fear noises. Eusebio never liked sudden noises or brusque movements, but he became much worse during those last years. I had to be explicit with friends and with anyone who came to the house warning them not to frighten him with a sudden appearance, not to speak too loudly behind his back, not to pat him on the arms or the back or his head. He became absolutely untouchable with his illness. He was never a physically demonstrative person, rarely showing his affection with hugs, except in our intimate moments. He didn't like people who had to be constantly touching, "invading" the person they were talking to — and there are people like that. All his life he was very measured in expressions of affection. Andrés Trapiello, a renowned writer also from León, says of his own people that they rarely demonstrate affection, that they find it hard to exteriorise their feelings and they even flee from those who try to impose affection on them, they flee or they feel ashamed of being sentimental. They have a hard shell around them in León. They don't like fuss. Miguel Delibes, another Spanish novelist, also said something similar about his own dour but resilient Castilian people. Eusebio was a good example of this, which in no way meant that he did not have feelings. He was always an extremely sensitive man. And I have to admit to having been the object, though very rarely, of Castilian scorn, initially perhaps when his parents found it hard to accept that their son was going to marry a non-Catholic. In those days, his mother would have preferred a Spanish girl of the same religion who was prepared to be a perfect housewife and not work outside the home as I did. However, she was big-hearted and soon realised that Eusebio wasn't in such bad hands after all, and she eventually admitted her error of judgement to me and I became accustomed to her somewhat austere tongue, realising that beneath her critical disposition lay a sound and generous woman.

I have already mentioned that Eusebio had taken to whistling the same song without ceasing. That was in the early stages of his illness. Several months later, he whistled very little. Then he would sometimes whistle that patriotic Cuban song, *Guantanamera* — what are you missing in Cuba, my love? His main expression, however, was silence. He never answered anything I asked him. He didn't say anything. Nothing at all. Was he forgetting how to speak, to form words? I know that this can happen with this illness. I must admit to having felt very lonely then. I think we all realise that you can feel lonelier in unresponsive company than if you are actually alone.

But there were other more physical symptoms, perhaps unrelated to the dementia. The episodes he suffered of diarrhoea and vomiting worried me. They left him weakened, yet he rarely complained of pain. There were days when he seemed almost moribund, but would then come round again. He lost so much weight that he was but a skeleton of what he had been, so thin were his arms and legs and his skin hung in strips around his thighs and stomach.

Then he was overcome by what to me was an irritating slowness, almost as though he were anaesthetised. By this, I mean for example, that after he had emptied his bladder in the morning, he would return to the bedroom and sit for hours, literally hours, on the edge of the bed as if in an absent state, or was he simply so mentally confused that he didn't know what he had to do, how to dress, how to wash, incapable of mustering the enthusiasm to do anything. At those times I would do all I could to induce him to move and go to the bathroom. "Yes, alright," he would say, "I'm going now", but he sat on like a stone statue, barely moving an eyelid. There was nothing I could do because I didn't have the strength to physically guide him and sometimes I threatened to bring in someone else to move him. It is amazing how much a sick body weighs when resisting, despite the amount of weight he had lost I found it frustrating to keep on repeating the same plea: "Come on, you can't spend the whole day in your pyjamas! It's almost lunchtime!" But, of course, he wasn't the slightest bit worried about being in his pyjamas or being late for lunch. Later, I had taken to shaving him because if he tried to do it alone he didn't do it properly and if he tried to dress by himself he would put his trousers on top of his pyjamas, he wouldn't have taken his false teeth out to wash them, or wash his face properly. But, as I say, he took no notice of me when I told him to go to the bathroom. He would sit lost in his world, unconscious of time, unconscious of how long he had been sitting there. His was a world of absolute slowness, a long parenthesis between one action and another, between sleeping and waking. It seemed that time took on another dimension.

He became like a baby, defenceless in a world that he barely understood. I thought he felt relatively happy and protected inside his own house and garden, surrounded by the objects he had known all his life. Yet I realise that defencelessness is one of the saddest things in the life of a grown man or a woman. It is difficult to imagine how it must be to find oneself in a situation which is unrecognizable. We could all become defenceless in our latter years. People who die with their mind and body *in situ*, particularly if they reach very old age, are frankly lucky. But to finish your days in a hospital bed attached to catheters, or confined to the same chair without being able to move, to feel bodily pain, sadness in your mind, to have to depend on someone else to feed you, to use the toilet, to wash, all that is tremendously sad and humiliating. However, it is the end of so many people although they don't wish it to be so. That slow diminishing of capacities has to be accepted and, where possible, accepted with humour. No-one knows what awaits them. Fortunately, one of the advantages of old age is that, in general, we learn to accept situations that we would never accept in our youth. It is important, as my mother would say, to count all the good things in your life and to feel grateful for them.

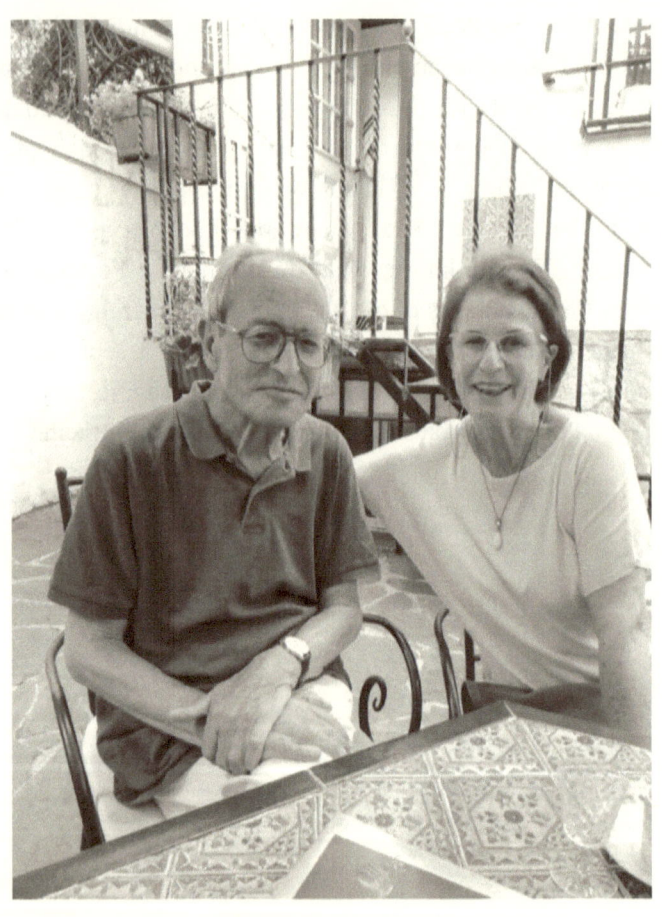

With Diana, July 2020

The Carer

How does Alzheimer's affect the person caring for their afflicted loved one? I suppose it's easier for a nurse or professional carer; someone generally much younger, and who can go home and forget the patient at the end of the day. The relationship is nonetheless complicated because the two people move at a different pace, the patient slowly without any apparent preoccupation, the carer quickly and with a thousand things to do. It is unnecessary to explain the frustration that the person in that role might feel. That person was me. I had to learn to arm myself with patience. I had to keep on saying that he no longer had the capacity to move more quickly. And it wasn't his fault.

Any carer needs respite. I had no intention of putting Eusebio in a Day Care Centre on a daily basis, but I did eventually succumb to doing this one day a week. And here is what I saw, though perhaps Eusebio did not. A spacious roomful of dilapidated human beings, mostly women, who couldn't hear, could barely see and whose bodies were like gnarled tree trunks, sagging around the roots. But it had come to this. Those hours gave me time to socialise, to relax and I used them to get out of the house, away from the daily routine and, from that point of view, it was a positive decision. However, the sentiments I experienced when I used to take him there and leave him, were hardly positive. I would walk him across the large lounge-cum-dining area at ten o'clock in the morning when some of the inmates were still having their breakfast, a hustle of trays and plates, cups and glasses of orange juice, a hustle to smother the silence of a hoard of old people who were incapable of communicating with each other. Any noise, apart from the dishes, came from the helpers who went briskly and sharply about their work, standing no nonsense — as I imagine they were paid very little for what they did, and certainly had no time to stand round talking to anyone.

I quickly realised that it was useless to ask them any questions and, of course, they were never there all day long. Those who worked at the breakfast round generally finished their shift mid-morning, when others took over and then again in the afternoon a new batch of helpers were there. There was a certain attempt at coordination between them, not always successful. Sometimes they had no idea if Eusebio had eaten well, if he had attended the physical exercise hour or his yoga in the afternoon. So the Day Centre was, for me, a combination of relief, frustration and depression. I felt so sad leaving him sitting defenceless in a chair beside these old people with whom he had no possibility of communicating, even if they had been able to communicate physically with him, because he was on a different mental plane to most of them. And when I went to pick him up in the early evening, they were all sitting round in front of a television emitting stupid, raucous programmes that none of them was in the least interested in.

It was a large centre, not only day centre, but a geriatric residence with all its unpleasant odours, even though it was exquisitely clean and the inmates seemingly well cared for, with pleasant receptionists and administrative staff. And so, despite my questioning the fairness of what I was doing by taking him there, we dropped into the routine. It meant a morning and evening walk for him of about a quarter of an hour each way. Every time he would ask me a good ten times where we were going. I used to tell him he was off to see the nurses at the Centre and he would retort, "No, No, No!" But continued walking all the same. And every time, I would say, "I shan't be long, I shall be back soon for you" and each day he would ask me what he had to do there and when was I coming back. But he took it all with a certain docility.

In fact, in a situation which wasn't always easy to cope with, his docility was something else for which I was grateful. You'll recall that during almost all his life, Eusebio had a quick temper with members of the family, sometimes with friends and with people he met along the way. Those outbursts of temper weren't always easy to manage, but I felt that they had to do with the fact that he considered that his ego had been attacked. He found it hard to put up with people if they had an opinion radically different to his. I think that, deep down, his strong reactions were because he was on the defensive and that they were the result of a basic insecurity in himself, in his place in society. They were brought on by a feeling of inferiority somehow innate in him, perhaps the result of the hardship of his early years, despite the success he had made of his career.

I think I have also mentioned that Alzheimer patients can suffer a radical change in their behaviour — for better or for worse. Calm people can turn aggressive, well-educated people can become vulgar in their behaviour and those who are aggressive can become docile. Without exaggeration, I believe that Eusebio underwent quite an acute change in personality. From being an often inflexible and intransigent person, he became extremely easy to manage; from having a quick temper, he turned very docile.

That situation, however, could obviously have altered. In fact, I began to notice his negative attitude to shaving, showering and dressing. He didn't seem to want my help. "Off you go!" he said, "Out, off you go!" Not nastily, but it was more his determination to do everything by himself. At that time, his negativity didn't tend to last too long. From the moment he decided to get out of bed until he finished washing and dressing, the process could take well over an hour. An hour when I had to be available if he needed me to help him. I would have preferred to do it all by myself because then we would have finished quickly, but I felt it preferable that he continue to do it and I know that he himself preferred it that way. But for me it was aggravating.

Ambling

It may well be my Anglo-Saxon roots, but I have never been a good "ambler". I don't have the Mediterranean art of walking slowly or ambling. When I go out for a walk I like to move quickly, with the urgent step, typical of my race, of someone going directly to a specific place and with the specific motive of exercising my body even though I am not actually in a hurry.

I generally was in a hurry when, for example, I would go shopping because I wanted to return home quickly, where I'd had left Eusebio by himself. However, I do admire the way the inhabitants of southern Europe amble on their walks. It seems that they have all the time in the world. They normally walk in the company of friends, perhaps giving their tongues more exercise than their legs. They are capable of sitting on benches in the shade for hours — those who have those hours, mainly the old age pensioners — chatting about everything and nothing, smiling and laughing. It gives the impression that these southern races are happy, always animated, as if the problems of the world have nothing to do with them. Yet this isn't true because, like everyone else, they have a thousand worries; worries about how to reach the end of the month, about their children, their work or lack of it, their complaints about politicians and a thousand etceteras. Exactly the same as anywhere else. But that time for *walking out*, in Spain, beneath the splendid light of a Madrid afternoon, would seem to animate people to be alive, it lifts body and soul, it stimulates a smile and warmth. I have said, it is an art and I can see a lot of beauty in it. It is as though they are all philosophizing, even though they may only be talking about what they are going to put on the table for supper. Eusebio used to go out and sit for hours on a bench in Arturo Soria, observing the passers-by, perhaps imagining their lives. Observing? That was before. Later on he didn't observe anything, at least he didn't appear to.

Sometimes we went out arm in arm. It saddened me to see how he walked precariously on those occasions. He was never a rapid walker, but he had always been agile and sure of himself. But then he stumbled, dragged his feet, tripped up and he moved very slowly, so slowly by my side. I felt as though I was pulling a heavy parcel or walking with someone twenty years older than he was. And so we never got very far, because if I tried to coax him to walk further than normal, he protested and had to sit down.

* * *

The first time I noticed this new fragility was during our holidays in south-west Spain in the Province of Huelva, in the town of Isla Cristina. Fortunately, we were close to the sea, but quite a way from the commercial centre and, as we aren't capable of living without the daily newspaper, we used to have to walk a long way to buy it. It was then that I realised how hard it was for him to walk because he had to sit down on every couple of benches to rest. Towards the end of our holiday I used to leave him in the coffee bar outside the hotel whilst I went flying off to get the paper. He didn't want to walk along the beach and he didn't want to swim. He has never been a keen swimmer, he was a country lad from the interior, but he used to enjoy diving in and out of the waves and would spend a long time in the water. But on that holiday, no. I realised that he simply wasn't at all well, although he didn't complain of any pain, only of fatigue, of visceral fatigue.

It was during those days that, without my knowing it, his colon cancer was nibbling away at him. As if it wasn't enough for one man to have this withering of the brain! A couple of weeks after returning from Huelva, he underwent an emergency operation and spent seventeen days with their nights in a bed in the Ramón y Cajal Hospital. That was where they gave him a colostomy bag, something that he never really understood and it was better that he didn't try to change it because when he did try, he got himself in a terrible mess with the resulting odour throughout the house. It was essential to close doors and open windows and use sprays, and I couldn't ask that of him. I think that from that point in time his mind also suffered and he became even more useless. While he was in the hospital, we had to stay with him day and night. My sister-in-law, Beni, helped me with her customary generosity and strength of character — we took it in turns to stay one night of every two — and Eloísa and Jaime also stayed when they could. The whole family made an effort. I never lacked help because I knew that at any moment I could call on family, on Emiliana, Ruth, Silvia here in Madrid and have contact over the telephone with those in León, Susa and Elisa, with Judith and Luis Alberto and, later on, with Naiara. I am truly grateful to them.

* * *

Returning, to the subject of our daily walks in the summer, though they were a little less frequent in the winter. This is where I suffered with my Anglo-Saxon nature, that desire — almost a vital necessity — to walk quickly and with an ulterior motive. It was really hard for me to have to sit beside Eusebio on a bench in Arturo Soria, even though it is a very pleasant street, and watch humanity passing by. I always felt that I could have been doing something more useful. However, I had to check myself, *is it not useful to accompany a sick person*? Of course it is. It is extremely useful. It is really an act of love, of tenderness and of patience. And being aware of that, despite my own limitations, was how I managed to overcome my impatience. Then I began to take him with me on errands, to the bread shop, the chemist, the post office, to the supermarket and, taking him with me meant that I could go more slowly, I was less anxious because I hadn't left him alone at home. I don't think he particularly enjoyed those outings. It was all the same for him to be sitting on his patio or inside the lounge at home. But the exercise was good for him and filled a little of that enormous space which was the emptiness of his mornings or afternoons.

I was very conscious that it wasn't worth forcing Eusebio to go outside in the street, to eat more, to walk around our garden so as to exercise his legs which were then painfully thin because he was losing body mass. I think the important thing was to leave him to do what he wanted. That coaxing is, above all, so that the carer feels she is *doing something for the patient*, when all he wants is to be left alone. That *doing something* is to alleviate the carer's own conscience. It is the desire to be the perfect carer. But no, when the carer has been his wife for so many years, it wasn't necessary to demonstrate anything either to the patient or to anyone else, not even to herself. What was important was simply to be there, a physical presence, in a sort of continuum, so that he was calm and felt cared for and loved. Just that, without any fuss.

One of the saddest aspects for me, as my partner's carer, was the mental distance between us. It was very gradual. It was like an apprenticeship to living a future situation, a circumstance that had not yet occurred but for which I was emotionally preparing myself, almost inexorably. Day after day I began to imagine what it would be like to live a solitary life within the same space where I had lived accompanied for years and years. As my questions remained unanswered, and my comments of any type fell onto waste land, I felt more and more alone in the presence of my companion's silences. His complete lack of reaction immersed me into my own world and I realised that, to be able to survive, I had no option but to search deeply into that world, whatever it was, so as not to drown in despair. In my case I was grateful for my interest in reading, writing, playing — very badly — the piano, and I was equally grateful to find pleasure in contact with others, well, in a controlled fashion.

I don't enjoy constantly chit-chatting with others, or being surrounded by a lot of people. I also needed that silence that was imposed on me by the situation. At our best times, Eusebio and I had shared lots of tasks, comments, observations of one sort or another and I recall that we used to talk at length into the small hours of the morning about the state of the world and about many other lesser things. We shared the same sense of humour. Our taste in films coincided, in books and even in music. Yet we never talked for hours without stopping about just anything at all. He had always been a serious man with weighty preoccupations and didn't enjoy stupidity, *absurdities* as he would say. His ecclesiastical education had prepared him for silence. He found much in society absolutely insufferable and that, together with his own sense of decorum, put a brake on his indulging in stupidities, not even "stupidities", but what he himself considered as nonsensical. That said, we had lived many hours together in silence. There are people who need incessant noise in the house, the radio, the television, music, whatever, to drown their own thoughts or maybe just because they cannot abide silence, that reunion with oneself. But that was never our case. I am perfectly capable of spending a whole day in silence, with my activities obviously, but I reserve my hours of television for the evenings.

It was those solitary activities and, more recently, I would add to the preferences already mentioned, the peace of mind that I find caring for the garden, that satisfied me. I rarely did the gardening when Eusebio used to do it. Yet now I feel a certain duty towards it, the duty of caring for his legacy, of not allowing it all to wilt and die. And all these things helped me to confront an extremely sad situation because, although I was perfectly conscious that death could come to me before it came to him, it seemed logical by age and illness that he go first. But no-one knows about such things. In any event, one of the two would have to leave the other and if I were the one left to stay in this world longer, I realised that I was in some way preparing myself for that moment.

It was difficult, if not impossible, that Eusebio could participate in anything that I did, in anything that I thought, in anything that I saw, not even in the colour of the flowers. Thus, against my will, I was forced to search for interests that fulfilled me even though I knew he was unable to share them with me. He sat, I moved; he slept or dreamed; I busied myself with the thousand tasks in the house and with my personal interests. That was the distance between us.

* * *

This illness wounds the heart with its cruelty. Or, is it not *cruel* when someone can barely remember anything about his life? I think that it is, it is very cruel. Particularly in our old age when we realise that we have lived far more than what is left to us to live and therefore our memories are extremely important. Perhaps you will ask, "And so what if the patient doesn't realise? Is that so bad?" And, of course, there is some truth in that. Yet I am speaking of an objective cruelty. That terrible fact of having an entire life blotted out, as though it had never existed. For me, as Eusebio's main carer, that was a most acute emotional burden. I began to ask myself, "...but what sense did his life have then, if he couldn't remember the child he was, the lover he was, the good and bad moments in his career, in his marriage, how he played his role as father to Eloísa and

Jaime?" A fairly strict father, I seem to recall. But they are the ones who should respond to that question.

The absolute self-centredness of a dementia patient is also difficult to manage for the person at his side. There was no gratitude for the attentions he received. It was all taken for granted. He didn't acknowledge the hours I spent helping him to dress, to shower, in preparing his meals and, yes, walking at his pace in the street. Yet of course, gratitude is elusive. One can feel gratitude but not know how to express it. Someone else maybe feels it less, yet is more overt, more effusive. Perhaps this depends on one's character and, as for taking things for granted, well, that is something we all do at times. It is when a person or an object is missing, that you become aware of the gratitude you felt.

The life of anyone who has to care for somebody during a long period of time is prone to fatigue, to boredom with a routine imposed by the patient, to depression and tension. Initially I noticed none of these things. I suppose it was, in a sense, a novelty playing the nurse. I have never in my already long life had to be constantly responsible for a sick person. After several years of it, however, I could feel myself tired at times, bored at times, depressed at times and tense at times. Yoga and relaxation helped, being able to rest completely for only five minutes when I felt the weight of the situation. I was grateful, although I am certainly no expert, to have learnt a little about the techniques to relieve the body and refresh the mind. I was also grateful for the many hours when I could communicate, by phone or in person, with Elo and Jaime, with the family and with my friends. I could find that relief recounting all that Eusebio did, everything that was inside me. Because you can't lock that medley of emotions inside yourself, they have to be allowed to escape into the air around you, leaving you purged until the next challenge.

However, one thing that I noticed was that for months I suffered episodes of lumbago and a pain in my right leg like sciatica. I found it difficult to go up and down stairs quickly because of that pain. That physical handicap was merely the physical expression, though, of the inner stress I was feeling, because it all disappeared several weeks after his death.

What I must admit, despite myself, is a thought that would infiltrate into my mind, a thought in the shape of a question. How far does love reach out? Is it possible to continue loving someone who gives you so much work to which you can see no end? And I answer that question affirmatively. Of course you can go on loving, because love is made up of so many different components and, whether we like it or not, one of them is to resist the blows, knowing that they come involuntarily. Love is not all enjoyment. It also has its doses of pain. There is pleasure in cultivating patience, even though you know that the person being cared for cannot appreciate it. This has nothing to do with martyrdom, something to do with duty and morale.

It was hard to continue loving my companion because he was no longer the person I had known during years and years of my life. But beneath that last facet of his nature, I knew that he was there and that, above all, I could never have abandoned him. Neither could I have passed the duty of that care to anyone else, not even to my children. I have always thought that it isn't fair to lay that weight on their young shoulders if I can avoid it. A little relief, yes, like the Day Centre so that I was able to have a few hours free of a complicated situation. But to search for professional help would only be the solution if I were unable to cope physically with him. I hoped that that would never occur. I wanted him to remain at home until his end, as long as the situation still had a certain dignity. All that is love.

The questions. Where is the justice in all this? Why him? How can this have happened to someone who was intelligent, ethical, courageous, far more than many? It is useless to ask these questions. But I do ask them. I didn't only ask: Why him? I also asked: Why me? What had I done in life to have this thrown at me? It is petty though.

It is petty to look for blame. I believe that injustice is meted out arbitrarily, without any specific design or in revenge for a fault committed. And although it is of slight consolation, I found some help by realising that what I was going through was painful and difficult, yet there were millions of others in the world going through many, many other situations far worse than mine. At the end of the day, is there any justice in this world of ours? Not often. Injustice is normal in society and also in nature. In most cases, it is those who are the most defenceless, the most miserable, the poor and unhappy who suffer both types of injustice, either with punishments unjustly applied, a life without hope or opportunity, or with tsunamis, volcanic eruptions, fires, floods and drought and, of course, illness. All that rampages through humanity, leaving man defenceless, a victim in the face of an uncertain destiny. And Eusebio was victim of one of the worst illnesses of our times, an illness that converted him into a puppet, abandoned to the will of others. I hoped, at least where I was concerned, not to have let him down.

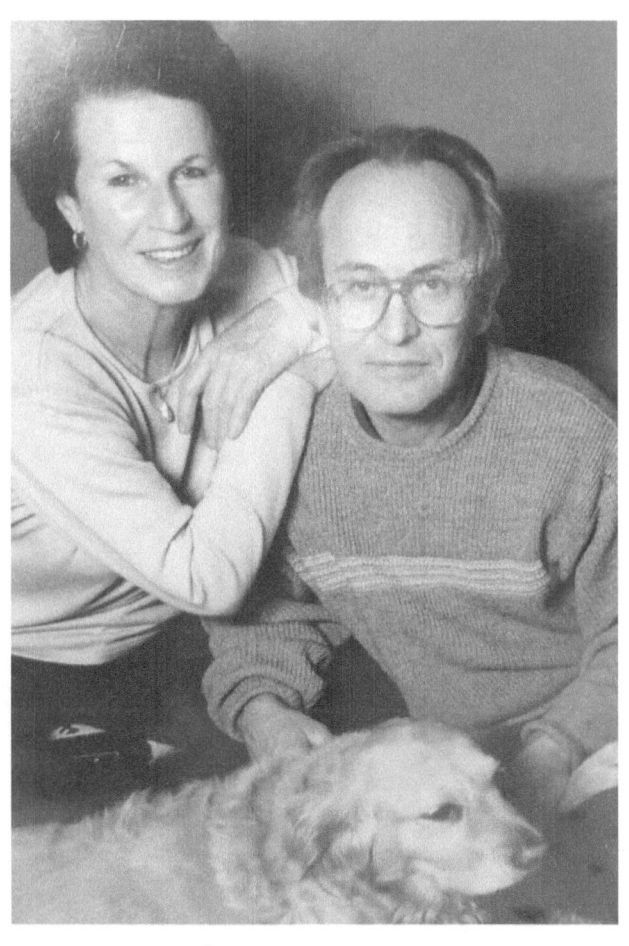

In our younger years

Medical Assistance

And what of the medical assistance that an Alzheimer patient receives? Those visits to the neurologists. Did they serve for anything? Very little, really, except perhaps in the beginning when he was given a brain scan to establish the cause of his memory failures, when it was evident that his neurones were dying in part.

Before consulting the specialists, however, there were several visits to his GP, a pleasant woman although seemingly austere in character and rather a teaser. It was obvious that she enjoyed asking Eusebio questions, playing the psychologist. She could see from that first visit that he wasn't well. She asked him about his profession and when she realised that he had spent years in politics, she asked him who the Prime Minister was and he answered, after slight hesitation, Felipe González. It was José Luis Rodríguez Zapatero at the time, but Eusebio remained with Felipe because he had been Prime Minister for almost all the years Eusebio had been a politician. I am saying that he had remained behind in time because his mind hadn't assumed the changes that had occurred between Felipe and the present. He could still tell the doctor his address. But he didn't remember what he had eaten for lunch that day, nor the date, nor the month, nor the year we were in. He simply said that those things didn't interest him and that was why he didn't remember them.

That visit to his GP was the start of a long series of visits to the neurologists. Frustrating it was, to say the least. I can swear that, with two visits annually, after some ten visits, we never saw the same neurologist. Of course I realise that the information about the patient is on the computer, that all Eusebio's data were there for the specialists to see. Yet I am not talking about data. I am talking about communication, about the personal knowledge that one or two neurologists might have had of him, about the fact that he himself might have been able to recognise his neurologist and that, although he forgot things and faces, he might have just had a little recognition for that person who was trying to help him.

I am speaking of Spain's National Health Service, but we have visited other specialists who were always the same every time we saw them, his urologist, his oncologist, the surgeon who operated his colon cancer, but for some strange reason that I have never understood, the neurologists appeared to take turns. One of them told me once that they formed a team of six neurologists. I can only say that we saw more than six of them. As a consequence, there was a sensation of uselessness about these visits. In fact, only a little while ago, as a result of the Covid-19 pandemic, a neurologist phoned telling me that it wasn't necessary for Eusebio to return to their consultancy unless he was suffering from an attack of some sort. She admitted that there was really no more they could do for him.

Obviously, they somehow had to reduce the number of appointments they received daily.

I could completely understand that, but it also confirmed the doubts I had had from the beginning, that those visits really served for very little. In fact, the last time we went after he had disappeared, she told me that it was unnecessary for him to continue with the medication as it was evident that it wasn't helping him, that it wasn't curing him and that it was no longer necessary. Better! Better for all of us! Tablets of any type may well cure a certain complaint, but sometimes, they induce some other complaint. In the long term at least, they may even be a danger for health, a waste of money.

I don't share that attitude in this society of taking medicines for anything at all and, although prevention may be better than cure, I certainly don't agree with so much preventive medicine. This is how the pharmaceutical industries earn vast quantities of money and very often they keep old people alive, yet in an appalling state. The only thing are pain-killers which help us to bear persistent or temporary pain, but to spend years taking pills ... just in case, no! However, informing us that they couldn't do any more for Eusebio, at least they were honest. It was a relief to be able to delete another medical appointment from the calendar. And so he wasn't taking any more medicine. They withdrew *Adiro* for blood clotting, *Atorvastatina* for cholesterol, and then *Ebixa* for Alzheimer's. Better. Much better! He continued to have a healthy diet. He ate very little and because he wasn't working, he didn't need much food to satisfy his energy requirements, or perhaps it was because of his cancer.

Then, in the latter months, the vomiting returned and, although he ate little and he had no bowel movements, his intestinal area swelled considerably. He never complained of pain, but he slept and slept, day and night. He didn't want to walk at all — the truth was that he couldn't, he had become so physically weak.

And so I found myself at a crossroads, of whether I should take him to hospital or not. Against taking him was the fear of contracting the Covid-19 virus. We had been advised not to go anywhere near medical centres as they were nests of possible contagion. I also asked myself what they would do for him, a few tests and home again with medicines after a few hours. I was against taking him also because he had no signs of pain, only that overwhelming fatigue, and so why cause him more disturbance by going out and embarking on a journey of injections, catheters, scans and the thousand other inconveniences of hospital life when he could remain tranquilly at home? But then, I thought, they might have been able to relieve him of the swollen diaphragm, induce him to evacuate all that was molesting him within and offer him any palliative care that he might need.

One never knows what is the right path to take. In his situation, everything was a risk, everything was advisable or inadvisable, everything required patience and a certain dignity.

The Final Weeks

When they told me that if I didn't decide to operate, he might have lived only another few days, my whole system fell into shock. Everything we had decided about no more operations, no more chemotherapy, seemed to collapse into a sea of cruelty. I even forgot that his life no longer had any quality. Was it to alleviate my own situation that I didn't want to operate? It was the inevitable battle, the eternal battle between mind and heart, between the rational and the emotional, whose solution could only be rash and drastic. And I began to reflect on the long hours of loneliness that awaited me — as if this was a relevant factor as to whether to operate or not. There is so much doubt in a decision of this nature. So I fought between the idea that I would be alleviating his suffering, which I knew was there, although unspoken, and the idea that I was not taking advantage of all the medical possibilities open to him.

A soul-searching dilemma. Surely that should have been a moment for writing truly beautiful things. Yet the stress and the noises and voices and movement, the sudden irruptions into the minute, airless cubicle of the emergency ward, all that was barely conducive to beauty and deep thoughts. The fatigue and exhaustion of having spent the night on a small, hard chair didn't help either.

I would look at his face and try to concentrate on our long past together, his beautiful face, free of wrinkles although his mouth was smothered behind the virus mask and a long tube emerged from his nose and his nightdress was slipping from his shoulders. Was it merely a question of letting him go with dignity? But there is no dignity in the dying process with tubes stuck up your nose, evacuating all your body fluids into plastic bags, being fed from other plastic bags with the liquid dripping through a catheter. Unaware he was, totally unaware of what surrounded him or what awaited him.

And several days later, more than a week later, after he had been transferred to a hospital bed in the cancer ward, we were still there waiting, waiting for Godot or for a miracle to occur. Both imaginary. After two days of almost brute strength and violent words, he seemed to have fallen back into a state of utter apathy. There was a lost indifference in his gaze, an all-pervading fatigue, an impossibility to muster enthusiasm for his 80 years. Again, the doctors asked us if we wanted to operate, not to extirpate but to pull the tumour aside to alleviate his blockage. A doctor in our family advised strongly against a further operation. He said that decisions like this were taken by a team of doctors who often only wanted to put their knowledge to practice without necessarily having the patient's well-being in mind. Is that indeed the case? We all only wanted him to go in peace and in dignity.

As for me, I experienced moments of great strength and times for tears to mitigate the profound sadness I felt at the idea of losing my companion of over 50 years. As yet, the full weight of the emptiness I was hurtling towards had not hit me. A page somehow had to be turned. I had lived in our home in solitude for a good three years, doing everything, all the house and garden, the banking, decision-making, completely alone except for that "other presence" and so the absence of that "other presence" was what I would be sure to notice, the agonising depth of a void because my soulmate would no longer be beside me. Courage! Is courage easier to muster, perhaps, at 75 than during the younger years? Maybe.

I was beginning to wonder if it wouldn't be long. He was weak, he no longer got agitated when he wanted to urinate, his voice was weakening, he slept and slept. He offered only a watery smile to the doctors and nurses in this pleasant hospital where he had been transferred to spend his final hours in palliative care. Apart from that, what was there? There was only his hermetic condition, an absolute withdrawal into himself. In one way, I feared it. I feared his thoughts, that he was perhaps aware we had taken him there to die, that he reproached me for not having done more to save him. I suppose that was my guilty conscience. I also found it frightening that a person doesn't have the need to communicate verbally, to share his thoughts with another. But in another way, I admired it. I considered him noble and strong inside his thoughts, his patience, his tolerance of his destiny, indeed, of the human destiny.

The end could be terrible after this long wait, because I had fallen into a sort of inertia when it was difficult to imagine how his end might occur. I even imagined that the days and nights would continue thus, interminably.

I am convinced that one of the benefits of old age is an easier acceptance of what life has in store for us. One can still feel rage for injustice in the form of warring, corruption, cruelty, untimely death, but the end seems easier to accept when one has run a good distance in life, when one has had "a good innings", as Eusebio and I have. It is pointless to rebel against death, however sad and infuriating its reality.

There were times when I felt that his end was approaching when I saw him so pale, so emaciated, so weak and so heavy with sleep. I tried as hard as I could to push that idea away, but it was inevitable and it hung in the air of his hospital room. Very often, when I tried to accept what was awaiting us, Eusebio would revive and begin to whistle, not the way he used to, neither as lively nor as strongly, but he whistled. And his complexion would take on a brighter colour.

Almost four weeks had passed and he was still resisting. Did anyone ever say that my dear husband wasn't a strong man? The answer to that is that he was really very strong, not only a strong heart, but also, and above all, a strong spirit. I believed that it was his inner strength that was keeping him alive rather than a robust heart. Yet he was sleeping more and more. He slept sitting. He slept lying down. He slept at night. He slept during the day. His indifference to everything around him was absolute. He didn't seem to realise whether he was accompanied or not. He still seemed to know us, within the remote folds of his memory, although he couldn't say our names or anything about us. When he saw us in photographs, he didn't sustain his gaze. Did he recognise that we had been part of his now unattainable past and he didn't like that? Did he know that he had no future?

A month passed. I have said that he had stamina, a stout heart, and above all, inner fortitude. There were times when I even doubted that perhaps he was as ill as they made out, that they exaggerated the time he could last out on serum only. But of course, they were administering pain-killers and tranquillisers so that maybe he seemed better than he really was and so that he could go towards his end in a painless and more dignified manner.

* * *

It is objectively sad sitting for hours beside someone waiting for him to die, yet subjectively, the quiet and tediousness of those long hours, which admittedly I interspersed with reading and TV and exercise in the room, represented a coming to terms with our life together and with his end and with my own future as a widow. I was in a sense thankful to have had that time to accept the future with a certain peace of mind and understanding, not to have had him ripped cruelly from my side without emotional preparation. I knew that until it actually happened, I wouldn't be aware of the full impact that his absence would have on my own life, on the lives of Elo and Jaime. But I was grateful for those moments to be able to do a little soul-searching. One of the strongest aspects for me about our marriage was the solidity that Eusebio had brought to it.

There was utter peace and tranquillity in his disposition. A seemingly complete absence of pain. They gave him palliative drugs: *Buscapina* against intestinal pain, *corticoids* against inflammation and an accumulation of phlegm, and *Paracetamol* to eliminate all types of pain. Perhaps there would still be other bad days when his mind would be turbulent and he would be ill at ease with his body, but I knew they were doing all possible to help him to leave this world in peace. And that is a beautiful word in his condition. I wanted him to find peace at the end of his life, for his journey over his eighty years had not always been happy and calm and confident. He found that society could be so irritating, so annoying. He deserved those last days of peace.

Yet, for me, it was hard to accept that he might not wake up again before his end. That was on his third day of sleeping. Would there be no more recognition? How tragic for his children. I didn't believe that the doctors knew when to expect his end. They didn't even seem particularly sure about his final symptoms, yet they have seen death approach so many patients. Or is it that they preferred not to be explicit for fear of upsetting me? Suddenly, I found myself wishing more fervently that the end would come soon. What more could we do? What more could we say? It was prolonging the agony in a state of pointlessness. Was it too much to ask that he gently drift from his state of somnolence to his death?

And in our silence, I told him that I loved him, that he had always been a courageous man, that he had planted not one tree, but twenty trees, that he had had not one child, but two, and that he had written not one book, but six or seven (the Cuban poet, José Martí, wrote that every man in his lifetime should have one child, plant one tree and write one book). I also told him that he had always been a solid, stable person, an anchor for me with my more voluble nature. That he had been a good man and that he had taught me to love this land, with its vast expanses in Castile, its Asturian mountains, its Mediterranean beaches, the beaches of Cadiz, and the Moorish architecture in Andalucía. I whispered those things to him, not too close to his ear because he never liked people molesting him or touching him. He never became accustomed to the nurses and doctors touching him, although he put up with it without protesting too much.

To sleep, to sleep and perhaps to dream. Whether 'tis nobler in the mind to suffer the slings and arrows of outrageous fortune, or to take arms against a sea of troubles ...I think that Eusebio did both. He was a determined fighter, yet he also suffered what he considered injustices on many an occasion. At times intransigent and over-sure of himself, inflexible and unseeing, in contrast acutely perspicacious, calm and solidly noble. Doses of good and bad, positive and negative. All of us are made up of good and bad, positive and negative and of many other facets.

And would that be his end, a gentle transformation from his deep sleep to his death? I hoped so. I waited anxiously, because I had never before accompanied anybody in that final transit. I had no idea at all how it would occur or how it would affect me, that finality. I would look at him and perhaps suddenly realise that his breathing had stopped, that the turbulent sounds and movements in his intestines had ceased, that the colour and texture of his skin had altered and then I would know that he was entirely, completely at peace. I desired that end for him. I had no wish to watch him suffer with agitated movements, with guttural breathing, with vomiting, with any sort of confusion or pain. I had already said that he deserved a peaceful death. He had always feared death — his Catholic upbringing perhaps. Could he not be shown that death was easy, painless, a diminishing of the life force, a fading away from things material, from loved ones, but to be in an immaterial place where there was no final judgement, no hell-fire, oblivion only. A long and lasting sleep. Rest at last from life's turmoil. I couldn't believe that this vital, agile, intelligent companion of mine was living out his last hours, barely able to move his skeletal frame, unable to utter any word, unable to concentrate on anything at all. Was this a cruel turn of fate? Objectively yes, but it was subjectively kind. His unawareness was the cloak that suffocated any feeling he might have had of fear, of inadequacy. He had already been gone from this world for a long time.

I felt bleak on that Sunday, horribly alone after so many days with him in the hospital. Earlier on, they had discovered cases of Covid-19 in the clinic and so from that day I was the only member of the family allowed to be with him. Again, I told myself not to be selfish, that many had it far worse. What did this have to do with the refugees in Lesbos, ousted from their temporary hovels by flames? I shouldn't complain. Yet there were long moments of introspection. Was it fair to allow him to continue in that state with all of us depressed, our lives in abeyance because it was impossible to live a normal routine, let alone undertake any new activity? Yes, we were existing in a limbo and it was a battle not to become embittered. A sensation of uselessness and doom spread its influence over my whole being to the point where I felt concerned about the future. Suddenly there was just no more to say to the nurses, to the doctors, to my loved one. And barely to friends or family. When a situation of that sort is perpetuated, boredom and inertia set in crushing imagination and initiative. That grey Sunday was doing that to me. Patience, Diana, patience!

Was it cruel to say that I didn't want him to continue for any longer in that state? It might have sounded cruel, but it wasn't. What I considered cruel was maintaining him in a condition devoid of hope and any possible future. Surely all they would have had to do was to have removed the drip and sedated him so that he would be unaware of hunger, thirst, pain or any other discomfort. I had reached the stage where I no longer felt grateful for the hospital's supposedly humane treatment. There was nothing humane in watching someone become weaker and more defenceless daily because he was being kept alive artificially. Yet I realised that what they were doing was the legally accepted way to treat his situation in Spain. And I had to look at my own conscience. How would I have felt if I had tried to force a decision to shorten his path? Justifiable only by claiming that I wanted to end his suffering. Was it perhaps to put an end to my own agony? How could I have lived with such a decision for the rest of my life? Eusebio was calm and not suffering, at least not evidently, so things should be allowed to take their natural course and I should have realised that those few weeks I was spending alone by his bedside were nothing in time when compared with a whole lifetime. As the doctor had said: Who were we to take life? Euthanasia/suicide is only justifiable when life is a torment. Again, who decides? These are not easy questions. Morality should not be lightly shunned.

Was it possible that I would miss that place when he died? I remembered the words in one of Eusebio's novels, *La Clínica*, about those who accompany patients and how the hospital can become an essential part of their existence to the point that they miss all the hours they spend at a bedside. I thought that I would miss those hours, not the hospital in itself, but the long time I was beside him. They excluded me from any other activity, yet I would miss him deeply in his absence which I would have to learn to fill in other ways, probably similarly to the way I always have, but there would be an immense void in my life when I would no longer be able to observe his beautiful face, the tranquillity of his expression, to hear the light snores coming from his mouth, to watch the rise and fall of his body beneath the bedclothes. Those days of emptiness were approaching and I would have to learn how to fill them. I would have to do some reorganising of my days. Eusebio had been my anchor, a guide in my life. He had calmed my volubility. He had kept me on the straight and narrow. And, above all, I loved him so profoundly.

We all hurt each other at times, without wanting to, each according to his nature. You hurt me. I hurt you. Yet, despite that, the love we felt had bound us in eternity.

* * *

And now that you aren't here — because you AREN'T here, hard as I find to believe that — all that is left to me is to say that I loved you so deeply. My wise owl. Nobody can even come up to your ankles. You, my love, were worth more than me. Why did you go first, leaving me with this profound pain?

You were untouchable. You only knew how to show affection in our intimate moments, of which there were many, but when I searched for your affection during the day, you would answer me with a brusque movement of your arm, something you would often do, yet with a teasing smile, and I would tell you to get lost, also with a smile. But these momentary displays of daily frustration are not important. We are like that. I only know that you were of gold.

You used to love pistachios, nuts, sunflower seeds, almonds, small fruits like grapes and cherries. I don't know what that was, because I always preferred the larger fruits like nectarines, oranges, peaches. Perhaps it came from the slow hours in your village when it gave you something to do in your youth, to peel the seeds and the pistachios, to break the shell of the walnuts, eliminate the seeds from the grapes, as you sat in the courtyard of your village home living out those lazy hours?

I have still said nothing of your death, of your final hours, when you couldn't get your breath and your breathing came rapidly in small, almost noiseless gasps. Then your eyes couldn't focus on my finger, and I knew that was the end. And that end lasted about four hours, painless I think for you and time enough for Eloísa to come and tell you that you were going to see our magnificent Catón, your parents, Francisco Umbral and Sartre and Camus, and many whom you had known and admired. And then the miracle occurred. At least for me it was a miracle. I don't know if you were trying to say goodbye to me, or thank me, or implore me to go with you. I don't know and I never will know. All I do know is that your face lit up with the most superlative light. You opened your eyes wide as I had never seen you do. You searched questioningly for my gaze and, at that moment, I told you how much I had loved you. What did you want to say, my love? Then there were a few small grunts as you attempted to rescue your last breath. And you went. Afterwards came the cold. The cold of your forehead, like marble, inert and lifeless. And so much pain!

However, I can truly say that to have accompanied you in your final hours, during the transit between your life and your death, was for me one of the most beautiful experiences that I have known in all my days. Because I had feared it so. I had never before been beside a moribund person. One of the most beautiful experiences, because I felt that I was accompanying you on your path towards peace, towards the absence of suffering, but also one of the saddest because of the immensity of the abyss that you would leave in my life.

*　*　*

Now, as I sweep up the autumn leaves in the garden, in our garden, in your garden which is mine now, I can feel your presence. You used to sit in the sun, between the two olive trees, then you would move to the shade. Sometimes you would watch me work. But you had given up and no longer wanted to help with a task which had been yours. But now I rescue your presence, the hours and hours you used to spend caring for your plants, for your trees, pruning their dead branches, encouraging them to grow with your love, an activity which replaced for you the hours you had dedicated to politics, to writing, to reading, because all that faded little by little in the autumn, the near winter of your life, my love. Yes, now in my hours of solitude, I rescue your presence there amongst your trees. Thank for that and for so much. Thank you for teaching me to love the lofty mountains of the north and south of this land, the beaches of the Mediterranean and Cadiz, the olive groves of Jaén and, yes, above all, the vast expanses of your beloved Castile.

Madrid, December 2020

www.ingramcontent.com/pod-product-compliance
Lightning Source LLC
Chambersburg PA
CBHW020328010526
44107CB00054B/2025